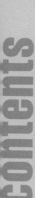

contents

24-hour clock

0000	12 midnight
0100	1 a.m.
0200	2 a.m.
0300	3 a.m.
0400	4 a.m.
0500	5 a.m.
0600	6 a.m.
0700	7 a.m.
0800	8 a.m.
0900	9 a.m.
1000	10 a.m.
1100	11 a.m.
1200	12 midday
1300	1 p.m.
1400	2 p.m.
1500	3 p.m.
1600	4 p.m.
1700	5 p.m.
1800	6 p.m.
1900	7 p.m.
2000	8 p.m.
2100	9 p.m.
2200	10 p.m.
2300	11 p.m.

Personal protective equipment (PPE)

- Wear *gloves* when there is a potential for soiling your hands with body fluids. Always wash your hands once you remove your gloves.
- Wear *goggles* when there is a potential for being splashed, splattered or sprayed with body fluids.
- Wear a *plastic apron* where there is a risk of bodily fluids contacting with your clothes.
- Wear a *mask* where there is the risk of inhaling or coming into contact with body fluids.

■ BODILY FLUIDS EXPOSURE

Step A *Immediately*
- Clean the area.
- If it is your skin, wash with soap and water.
- If it is a mucous membrane (e.g. eye), wash with water or saline.
- If it is a sharps injury, wash with soap and water.

Step B
- Report the exposure to your mentor or nurse in charge once you have completed Step A

Step C
- Adhere to the area protocol. This may involve presenting to either the emergency department of a hospital or a general practitioner.

Step D
- Record the incident on the organisation's adverse incident report form.

Medication administration

■ FIVE RIGHTS AND THREE CHECKS

FIVE RIGHTS	THREE CHECKS
• Right patient • Right medicine • Right dose • Right time • Right route *Note* also the right to refuse (under some circumstances)	• Check the label when getting the drug from storage. • Check the drug label with the drug chart. • Recheck the drug chart and drug after dispensing but prior to administration.

Medication administration is more than the five rights; it is about ensuring patient needs are met, that medicines have the desired effect, and safe outcomes result.

Commonly used and understood abbreviations for routes

Abbreviation	Meaning	Abbreviation	Meaning
PO	per oral/by mouth	IT	intrathecal
		PR	per rectum
NG	nasogastric	PV	per vagina
SL	sublingual	Gutt	eye drop
IV	intravenous injection	Top	topical
		MA	metered aerosol
IM	intramuscular injection		
SUBCUT	subcutaneous	Neb	nebuliser

Reference / Australian Council for Safety and Quality in Health Care (2005) *National Inpatient Medication Chart Guidelines.* Sydney: Australian Council for Safety and Quality in Health Care, p. 9. Reproduced with permission.

■ TIPS IN PREVENTING MEDICATION ERRORS

- Check allergies (ask patient, check for allergy band, check medication chart).
- Follow the five rights.
- Be certain of patient identity.
- Look up medicine in British National Formulary (BNF).
- Know therapeutic use of medication, normal dose, side effects and contraindications.
- Check expiry date.
- Check decimal points.
- Check measurement.
- Check the patient by name and arm band, and verbally if able.
- Don't guess the name if you cannot read it.
- Don't administer medication that is spelt or written incorrectly.
- Always question large doses.
- In paediatric patients, check weight/recommended dose and confirm with a second nurse.
- Students ALWAYS seek direct supervision by a Registered Nurse when administering medications.
- Don't leave medications on over-bed lockers/tray tables.
- Don't administer anything that you have not prepared yourself.

ALWAYS SEEK CLARIFICATION IF UNSURE.

■ SAFETY TIPS WITH ORAL MEDICATIONS

- Check the five rights.
- Ensure that you are directly supervised if you are a student.
- Make sure the patient is sitting up.
- Explain to the patient what the medication is.
- If dealing with children, seek their cooperation as well as that of their parents/caregivers.
- Make sure the patient is capable of swallowing.
- Check the patient has fluid to swallow the medication.
- When measuring oral liquid medicine do so at eye level, with the measure cup on a flat surface.
- Document appropriately.

- Don't give oral medication if the patient is:
  — sedated
  — has no gag/swallowing reflex
  — is vomiting.
- Check the patient for medication effect.

■ SAFETY TIPS WITH INJECTIONS

- Check the five rights.
- Ensure that you are directly supervised if you are a student.
- Be aware of onset of action and side effects.
- Know the landmarks for intramuscular (IMI) and subcutaneous.
- Use the correct needle and syringe.
- Never recap a needle.
- Dispose of the needle and syringe appropriately.
- Document appropriately.
- Check the patient for medication effect.

■ ABBREVIATIONS USED IN MEDICATION ADMINISTRATION

ac	before food	qh	every hour
bd	twice daily	q2h	every two hours
c	with	q4h	every 4 hours
gtt	drops	q6h	every 6 hours
mane	morning	q8h	every 8 hours
mist	mixture	stat	immediately
nocte	night	tds ⎫	
pc	after meals	tid ⎭	three times daily
prn	as required	ung	ointment
qid ⎫		unit(s)	International Unit(s)
qds ⎭	four times daily		

Reference / Adapted from Galbraith, A., Bullock, S. and Manias, E. (2004)
Fundamentals of Pharmacology, 4th edn. Sydney: Pearson Education, p. 935.
Reproduced with permission.

Every medication order should include:

- date
- route
- generic drug name
- dose ordered
- frequency
- time
- medical officer's signature

The medication chart should include:

- patient's name
- Hospital number
- date of birth
- address
- allergies
- weight

■ METRIC SYSTEM AND SYMBOLS

Metric system

VOLUME

1 litre (L)	=	1000 millilitres (mL)

MASS

1 kilogram (kg)	=	1000 grams (g)
1 gram (g)	=	1000 milligrams (mg)
1 milligram (mg)	=	1000 micrograms (µg)

LENGTH

1 kilometre (km)	=	1000 metres (m)
1 metre (m)	=	100 centimetres (cm)
1 centimetre (cm)	=	10 millimetres (mm)

EXAMPLE OF EQUIVALENCES

0.2 kilograms	=	200 grams
0.2 grams	=	200 milligrams
0.2 milligrams	=	200 micrograms
0.2 litres	=	200 millilitres

Decimals, percentages and fractions

DECIMALS	PERCENTAGES	FRACTIONS
0.01	1%	1/100
0.05	5%	5/100
0.20	20%	20/100
0.30	30%	30/100
0.40	40%	40/100
0.50	50%	50/100
0.60	60%	60/100
0.70	70%	70/100
0.80	80%	80/100
0.90	90%	90/100
1.00	100%	100/100

■ DRUG CALCULATIONS

Drug dosages

$$\text{Amount required} = \frac{\text{strength required}}{\text{strength in stock}} \times \frac{\text{volume}}{1}$$

OR

$$\text{Amount required} = \frac{\text{required strength}}{\text{stored strength}} \times \frac{\text{volume}}{1}$$

Intravenous infusions

Rate (drops per minute) = $\dfrac{\text{volume to be infused}}{\text{time in hours}} \times \dfrac{\text{drop rate}}{60 \text{ minutes}}$

(The drop rate is found on the drip set in the UK:
Macrodrop 20 drops/mL, Micorodrop 60 drops/mL.)

$$\text{Rate (mL/h)} = \frac{\text{volume (mL)}}{\text{time (hours)}}$$

µg/kg/min: this calculation is a three-step process

$$\frac{\text{ordered dose in µg}}{\text{volume (mL)}} \times \frac{\text{infusion rate (mL/h)}}{60} \times \frac{1}{\text{body weight (kg)}}$$

■ DRUG NAME ENDINGS AND RELATED INFORMATION

SUFFIX	DRUG GROUP	EXAMPLE
Anaesthetics (local)		
-caine	Esters	Procaine
		Amethocaine
	Amides	Lidocaine
		Prilocaine
Antibiotics		
-illin	Penicillin group	Ampicillin
-cycline	Tetracycline group	Doxycycline
-mycin	Macrolide group	Erythromycin
-oxacin	Quinolones	Ciprofloxacin
Cardiac/Antihypertensive drugs		
-olol	Beta blockers	Propranolol
-dipine	Calcium channel blockers	Felodipine
		Nifedipine
		Amlodipine
-pril	Angiotensin converting enzyme (ACE) inhibitors	Ramipril
		Lisinopril

SUFFIX	DRUG GROUP	EXAMPLE
-sartan	AT_1-receptor blockers	Losartan Irbesartan
Diuretics		
-ide	Loop diuretic	Furosemide
Fibrinolytics		
-inase	Enzyme	Streptokinase Urokinase
Neuromuscular blockers		
-ium	Depolarising or non-competitive blockers	Suxamethonium
	Competitive blockers	Atracurium Pancuronium
Oral hypoglycaemics		
-ide	Sulfonylureas	Gliclazide Gilbencalmide
Sedatives/Anxiolytics		
-azepam	Benzodiazepines	Temazepam Diazepam

■ DRUGS UTILISED AS ANTIDOTES

DRUG	ANTIDOTE
Benzodiazepine	Flumazenil
Paracetamol	Acetylcysteine
Warfarin	Vitamin K_1
Atropine	Physostigmine
Heparin	Protamine sulphate
Anticholinesterase	Atropine
Iron poisoning	Desferrioxamine
Narcotic	Naloxone
Digoxin	Atropine, phenytoin

Reference / Galbraith, A., Bullock, S. and Manias, E. (2004) *Fundamentals of Pharmacology*, 4th edn. Sydney: Pearson Education, p. 201. Reproduced with permission.

Oxygen concentration delivery

Nasal prongs: deliver a variable concentration of oxygen depending on respiratory rate.
With normal breathing:
2L oxygen minute will deliver 28%.
4L oxygen minute will deliver 35%.

Hudson mask

6L oxygen minute will deliver approx. 45%.
8L oxygen minute will deliver approx. 55%.
10L oxygen minute will deliver approx. 60%.
12L oxygen minute will deliver approx. 65%.
15L oxygen minute will deliver approx. 70%.

Non-rebreather mask

15L oxygen minute will deliver 85–100%
    (bag must be inflated).

OXYGEN FLOW RATE (L/MIN)		APPROXIMATE PERCENTAGE OXYGEN
NASAL PRONGS	2	28
	4	35
HUDSON MASK	6	45
	8	55
	10	60
	12	65
	15	70
NON-REBREATHER MASK	15	85–100 (bag must be inflated)

Fluid balance

■ MEASUREMENTS USEFUL FOR FLUID BALANCE CHARTS

1 jug	=	1000 mL
1 cup	=	250 mL
1 tablespoon	=	15 mL
1 dessertspoon	=	10 mL
1 teaspoon	=	5 mL

■ TIPS WITH FLUID BALANCE CHARTS

- If output is > intake, the patient is in a negative balance.
- If intake is > output, the patient is in a positive balance.
- Make sure patients know they have on a fluid balance chart.
- Always ask the patient their intake and output when updating the fluid balance chart.
- The urinary output should be >0.5 mL/kg/h (approx. 30 mL/h or 240 mL/shift).
- Report urinary output of <30 mL/h.
- Gain or loss of 1 kg equates to 1 L of fluid retained or lost.
- Positive or negative balances greater than 500 mL should be reported.

■ TYPES OF IV FLUIDS

- *Isotonic solution* has the same osmotic pressure as the body plasma. Isotonic solutions are:
  — whole blood
  — Hartmann's
  — 4% glucose with 0.18% sodium chloride
  — 5% glucose
  — 0.9% sodium chloride.

- *Hypotonic solution* has less osmotic pressure than plasma. Hypotonic solutions are:
  — water
  — 0.45% sodium chloride
  — 4% glucose.

- *Hypertonic solution* has more osmotic pressure than plasma. Hypertonic solutions are:
  — 25% mannitol
  — 10% glucose
  — 5% to 10% glucose combined with 0.2% to 0.9% sodium chloride
  — 20% albumin
  — gelofusine.

Reference / Adapted from Galbraith, A., Bullock, S., Manias, E., Hunt, B. and Richards, A. (2008) *Fundamentals of Pharmacology: An Applied Approach for Nursing and Health*, 2nd edn. Sydney: Pearson Education. Reproduced with permission.

Drip rates for giving sets where:
20 drops = 1 mL

1000 mL	mL/HR	DROPS/MIN
q2h	500	167
q4h	250	83
q6h	167	56
q8h	125	42
q10h	100	33
q12h	83	28
q16h	63	21
q24h	42	14

Vital signs

- Temperature (T): normal 36.5–37.1 PO
- Heart rate (HR): rate, rhythm, strength
- Respiratory rate (RR): rate, depth, pattern, use of accessory muscles
- Blood pressure (BP)
- Mean arterial pressure (MAP): {(systolic BP – diastolic BP)/3} + diastolic BP
- Blood saturation as measured by pulse oximeter (SpO_2)

Normal ranges

AGE (YEARS)	RESPIRATORY RATE (BREATHS/MIN)	HEART RATE (BEATS/MIN)	SYSTOLIC BLOOD PRESSURE (mm Hg)	SpO_2
<1	30–40	110–160	70–90	>98%
2–5	25–30	95–140	80–100	>98%
6–12	20–25	80–120	90–110	>98%
Adult	12–20	60–100	100–130	>98%

Note *This should be used as a guide only. Validation of parameters should be determined based on organisation policy.*

Reference / Mackway-Jones, K. (ed.) (2001) *Advanced Paediatric Life Support: The Practical Approach*, 3rd edn. London: BMJ Books. Reproduced with permission.

Quick head-to-toe assessment

General

Always provide privacy, compare right and left sides, and document and report findings.

Neurological

Look for signs of orientation to time and place.
Record Glasgow coma score (GCS) as necessary.

Glasgow coma score

SCORE	<4 YRS	4–15 YRS	ADULT
EYE OPENING			
4	Spontaneously	Spontaneously	Spontaneously
3	To verbal stimuli	To verbal stimuli	To speech
2	To pain	To pain	To pain
1	No response to pain	No response to pain	No response to pain
BEST MOTOR RESPONSE			
6	Spontaneous or obeys verbal command	Obeys verbal command	Obeys verbal command
5	Localises to pain or withdraws to touch	Localises to pain	Localises to pain

SCORE	<4 YRS	4–15 YRS	ADULT
4	Withdraws from pain	Withdraws from pain	Withdraws from pain
3	Abnormal flexion to pain	Abnormal flexion to pain	Abnormal flexion to pain
2	Abnormal extension to pain	Abnormal extension to pain	Abnormal extension to pain
1	No response to pain	No response to pain	No response to pain
BEST VERBAL RESPONSE			
5	Alert, smiles, babbles, coos words to usual ability	Orientated and converses	Oriented to time and place
4	Fewer than usual words, spontaneous irritable cry	Disorientated and converses	Disorientated and converses
3	Cries only to pain	Inappropriate words	Inappropriate words
2	Moans to pain	Incomprehensible sounds	Incomprehensible sounds
1	No response to pain	No response to pain	No response to pain

Reference / Adapted from Knight, G. J. and Slater, A. J. (2005) in Bersten, A. D., Soni, N. and Oh, T. E. (eds.) *Oh's Intensive Care Manual,* 5th edn. Edinburgh: Butterworth Heinemann, p. 1055. Reproduced with permission from Elsevier.

Cardiovascular
- Look at the patient's colour.
- Feel the distal pulses (radial, brachial, pedal pulses) and apical pulse (use stethoscope).
- Feel strength, rhythm and rate of the pulse.
- Feel for oedema in the feet and dependent areas.
- Obtain the blood pressure.

Respiratory
- Look for respiratory pattern, rate, symmetry, use of accessory muscles and patient position. (Does the patient look comfortable breathing?)
- Listen for equal air entry to both lungs.
- Listen for noises such as crepitations or wheezes.
- Examine the sputum.

Skin
- Look at the colour, scars or lesions.
- Feel the temperature, moisture, turgor, oedema and capillary refill (normal = <3 seconds).

Abdomen
- Look, then listen and then feel.
- Look for distension and scars.
- Listen for bowel sounds (normal sounds occur every 15–20 seconds).

- Percuss:
  — Dullness is a solid organ.
  — Tympany is air-filled.
  — Flatness is muscle or bone.
- Feel for pulsations, masses, tenderness and rigidity.
- Always start in the least painful area.

Extremities

- Look at the colour, movement, warmth, sensation and strength of limbs.
- Feel for swelling or pain in the calf caused by dorsiflexion of foot (Homans' sign). This may be an indication of thrombosis or thrombophlebitis in the leg veins.
- Look at nail beds for capillary refill or signs of clubbing and discolouration.

Other

Listen to the history of presenting condition:
- date and time of onset
- causative factors
- action taken to relieve symptoms
- family history
- medications
- social history, employment and family situation
- lifestyle, diet, alcohol and exercise.

Pain assessment

When assessing pain, remember PQRST:

Ask the patient:

P = *Precipitation/Palliation*   what causes the pain?
what relieves the pain?

Q = *Quality*   what does the pain feel like?
(is it sharp, stabbing, dull,
crushing)

R = *Region/Radiation*   where did the pain start?
where does the pain travel to?

S = *Severity*   how bad is the pain?
(use a pain scale: 0 = no pain,
10 = worst pain)

T = *Timing*   when did the pain start?
how long does the pain last?

Reference / Adapted from Ramont, R. P. and Niedringhaus, D. M. (2004) *Fundamental Nursing Care*. Upper Saddle River, New Jersey: Pearson Education, page 333.

Referred pain

AREA OF REFERRED PAIN	ORGAN
Neck, L. jaw, L. arm, upper back	Heart
L. shoulder	Lungs
L. shoulder	Diaphragm
R. shoulder, R. side	Liver
R. sided back pain	Spleen
Epigastric region, middle back	Stomach
R. and/or L. flank pain	Kidney
L. hypochondriac region, LUQ	Pancreas
Umbilical region	Gall bladder
R., L., or both inguinal regions	Ovaries
R. inguinal region, RLQ	Appendix
R. & L. inguinal regions	Ureters
Suprapubic, posterior gluteus/thigh	Bladder

L = left
R = right
LUG = lower upper quadrant
RLQ = right lower quadrant

Reference / Adapted from Ramont, R. P. and Niedringhaus, D. M. (2004) *Fundamental Nursing Care.* Upper Saddle River, New Jersey: Pearson Education, page 326.

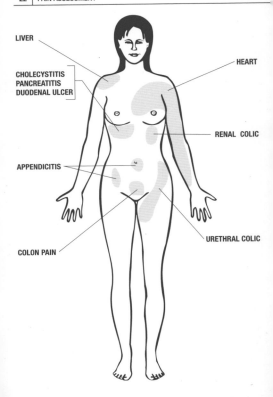

LIVER

CHOLECYSTITIS
PANCREATITIS
DUODENAL ULCER

HEART

RENAL COLIC

APPENDICITIS

URETHRAL COLIC

COLON PAIN

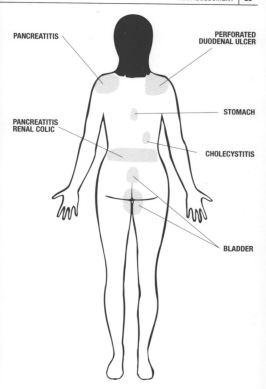

PANCREATITIS

PERFORATED
DUODENAL ULCER

STOMACH

PANCREATITIS
RENAL COLIC

CHOLECYSTITIS

BLADDER

Atomic symbols

Ca	Calcium
C	Carbon
Cl	Chloride
H	Hydrogen
Mg	Magnesium
O	Oxygen
K	Potassium
Na	Sodium
PO	Phosphate
HCO_3	Bicarbonate

Blood values

Cardiac enzymes

Note These normal adult values are a typical range and are relative to the type of test, equipment used and weight of patient. They are for guide only.

CARDIAC MARKERS				
MARKER	**NORMAL LEVEL**	**ONSET**	**PEAKS**	**DURATION**
Creatinine kinase (CK)	M: 55–170 u/L F: 30–135 u/L	3–6 hours	12–24 hours	24–48 hours
CK-MB	<5% of total CK activity	4–8 hours	18–24 hours	72 hours
Troponin (cTn)	Variable depending on methodology	2–4 hours	24-36 hours	7–10 days

Electrolytes

Sodium (Na)	134–146 mmol/L
Potassium (K)	3.4–5.0 mmol/L
Chloride (Cl)	98–108 mmol/L
Bicarbonate (HCO$_3$)	22–29 mmol/L
Anion gap	8–16 mmol/L
Osmolality calculated	275–295 mmol/L
Glucose	3.0–7.8 mmol/L; 3.9–6.2 mmol/L (fasting)
Urea (age-dependent)	4.0–8.0 mmol/L
Creatinine (age-dependent)	0.05–0.12 mmol/L (50–100 μmol/L)
Protein total	63–78 g/L
Albumin	35–45 g/L

Globulin	25–45 g/L
Bilirubin total	3–17 μmol/L
Alkaline phosphatase (ALP) (age-dependent)	35–150 U/L
Gamma—GT (GGT)	5–40 U/L
Alanine transaminase (ALT)	1–45 U/L
Aspartate transaminase (AST)	1–36 U/L
Calcium (Ca)	2.15–2.60 mmol/L
Calcium (alb. Corr.)	2.15–2.60 mmol/L
Phosphate (PO)	0.80–1.40 mmol/L
Magnesium (Mg)	0.70–1.10 mmol/L
Triglycerides	<200 mg/dL; <2.0 mmol/L (fasting)
Low-density lipoprotein (LDL)	<80 U; 2.0–3.4 mmol/L (fasting)
High-density lipoprotein (HDL)	>35 mg/dL; 0.9–2.2 mmol/L (fasting)
Total cholesterol	<200 mg/dL; <5.5 mmol/L (fasting)

Note Variations may occur depending on the age and sex of the patient.

Blood gases

pH	7.36–7.44
pCO_2	36–44 mmHg (4.5–6.0 KPa)
PaO_2	85–100 mmHg (11.3–13.3 KPa)
Bicarbonate	22–29 mmol/L
Base excess	−2 to +2 mmol/L
Oxygen saturation	94–98%

Thyroid function test

TSH	1–11 mU/L

Drug levels

Digoxin	toxic	>2 μg/L
	normal	1–2 μg/L
Paracetamol	toxic	30 mg/L
	normal	5–25 mg/L

Haematology

WBC	Age-related	$4.5–11 \times 10^9$/L
RBC	Age-related	Male $4.6–6.2 \times 10^9$/L
		Female $4.2–5.4 \times 10^9$/L
Hb		Male 130–180 g/L
		Female 120–160 g/L
Hct		Male 45–54 mL/dL
		Female 37–47 mL/dL
MCV		80–100 fL
Platelets		$150–400 \times 10^9$/L
Lymphocytes		25–33%
Monocytes		3–7%

Note Variations may occur depending on the age and sex of the patient.

Normal values in a routine urinalysis

pH	4.6–8.0
Specific gravity (SG)	1.003–1.030
Protein	<0.15g/day
Blood	up to 2 RBCs
Glucose	nil
Ketones	nil
Osmolality	38–1400 mOsm/kg H_2O

Reference / All material in the Blood Values section adapted from Knight, G. J. and Slater, A. J. (2005) in Bersten, A. D. and Soni, N. and Oh, T. E. (eds.) *Oh's Intensive Care Manual*, 5th edn. Edinburgh: Butterworth Heinemann; Harris, P., Nagy, S. and Vardaxis, N. (2006) *Mosby's Dictionary of Medicine, Nursing and Health Professionals*. Chatsworth, Australia: Elsevier; Wagner, K., Johnson, K. and Kidd, P. (2006) *High Acuity Nursing*. Sydney: Pearson Education.

Mental health assessment

It is very important that you gather as much information as possible in your initial assessment of the patient. To do this you need to develop trust and rapport with the person quickly. Be personable and ask open-ended questions. These will elicit the most information. You need to gather information under the following broad headings:

Personal—identifying information

- Name
- Gender
- Next of kin/Significant other
- Medications
- What does the person see as the presenting problem?
- Age
- Occupation
- Cultural affiliation
- Previous treatment

Appearance—person's physical presentation

- Grooming
- Posture
- Make-up
- Hygiene
- Tattoos/Piercing
- Other
- Clothes
- Scars

Mood—variability, intensity and appropriateness

- Worried
- Tearful
- Angry
- Elated
- Irritable
- Scared
- Flat
- Hopeless
- Labile

Behaviour—behaviour exhibited/context

- Calm
- Tremors
- Facial movements
- Attitude
- Hyperactive
- Agitated
- Rigid
- Aggressive
- Inappropriate
- Gestures
- Language used
- Suspicious

Perception—check the five senses (visual, auditory, tactile, olfactory, taste)

- Hallucinations
- Illusions

Thoughts—processes and content observed in conversation

- Delusions (false beliefs)
- Phobias (what?)
- Paranoia (who & what?)
- Tangential thoughts
- Concrete thoughts
- Obsessions (about?)
- Blocking
- Other

Safety—ask direct questions

- Suicide: Are you thinking of hurting yourself—how?/when?
- Homicide: Are you thinking of hurting someone else—who?/how?/when?

Memory—brief cognitive assessment

- Orientation
- Concentration
- Alertness

Insight and judgement—person's awareness about condition and decision making

- Ask patient about nature of the illness. Is self-assessment realistic/unrealistic?
- Ask such questions as 'What would you do if you saw an old lady lying on the road?'.
- Explore patient's impulse control.

Check information with relatives and other staff who may know the person. Avoid being confrontational, give the person an explanation as to what you are doing and be aware of your own biases, attitudes and judgemental behaviour. Write up notes quickly in an objective, professional manner noting context of assessment and persons present.

Resuscitation

■ CARDIAC RHYTHMS

Sinus rhythm

Sinus rhythm is the normal rhythm of the heart and consists of the following wave formations.

P wave	represents contraction of the atria
PR interval	should be no greater than 0.2 seconds or 5 small squares
QRS complex	represents contraction of the ventricles and should be no wider than 0.12 seconds or 3 small squares
T wave	is the resting phase of the heart

Electrocardiogram (ECG) paper

- Time is measured on the horizontal axis.
- Voltage is measured on the vertical axis.
- Each small square = 0.04 seconds.
- 1 large square (5 small squares) = 0.2 seconds.

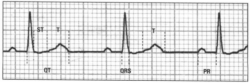

To calculate rate

Count the number of large squares between two R waves and divide 300 by this number

Reference / From Yang, K., Foote, S. and Janz, K. F. (2004) *ECG Interpretation for Exercise Testing*. Iowa City: University of Iowa, as requested by K. F. Janz. Reproduced with permission.

Usual waveform of an ECG

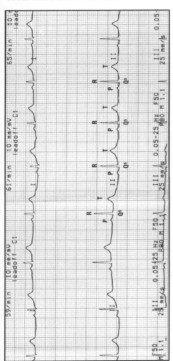

■ WHEN TO SEEK HELP

AREA	SIGNS AND SYMPTOMS FOR ADULTS
AIRWAY	Threatened airway (i.e. person having difficulty breathing, or noisy breathing)
BREATHING	• Use of accessory muscles or sternal recession • Respiratory rate <12 or >25 breaths/minute • SpO$_2$ of less than 95% • Respiratory arrest
CIRCULATION	• A change in HR of 20 beats a minute from the patient's baseline parameters or a pulse rate <50 or >120 beats/minute • A change in BP of 20 mmHg from the patient's baseline parameters or a systolic blood pressure <90 mmHg • Cardiac arrest
NEUROLOGICAL	• Sudden fall in consciousness or difficult to arouse • Fall in the Glasgow coma scale of >2 points • Seizures
OTHER	• Any person you are concerned about

ALWAYS SEEK HELP SOONER RATHER THAN LATER.

■ CPR

CPR for cardiopulmonary resuscitation.

	AIRWAY	COMPRESSION	
			1 or 2 people
INFANTS <1 YEAR	Normal position of head. Chin lift or jaw thrust if necessary. Do not overextend neck tilt	2 fingers Lower third of sternum	30:2
YOUNGER CHILD: 1–8 YEARS	Chin lift or jaw thrust; head tilt more than infants but less than adults	heel of one hand Lower third of sternum	30:2
OLDER CHILD: 9–14 YEARS	Chin lift, jaw thrust or head tilt	2 hands Lower third of sternum	30:2
ADULT	Chin lift, jaw thrust or head tilt	2 hands	30:2

Note Division between children above and below 8 years no longer occurs in the UK resuscitation guidelines.

Rate of compression
100 compressions/minute

Depth of compressions
Adult/child/infant: ⅓ of the depth of the chest (4–5 cm in adult)

Position of hands
Adult/child/infant: Middle of the lower half of sternum or centre of chest

Inspiratory time
1 sec to produce chest rise as in normal breathing

Common emergency drugs: dose and action
1 ADRENALINE
Use: First-line drug; ventricular arrhythmias with no cardiac output or low cardiac output states (VT, VF, PEA, asystole)

Dose: 1 mg IV repeated every 3–5 minutes if VF/VT persists

Action: Peripheral vasoconstriction directing available cardiac output to myocardium and brain

2 ATROPINE
Use: Symptomatic slow heart rates

Dose: 1 mg repeated to a maximum of 3 mg

Action: Parasympathetic antagonist; increases the heart rate

3 AMIODARONE

Use: Ventricular arrhythmias (VT, VF, SVT) or following failure of defibrillation and adrenaline

Dose: 300 mg bolus, additional 150 mg may be considered followed by an infusion of 900 mg over 24 hours

Action: Class III antiarrhythmic

4 LIDOCAINE

Use: Ventricular arrhythmias (VT/VF) or failure of defibrillation and adrenaline, if amiodarone is unavailable

Dose: 1 mg/kg bolus

Action: Antiarrhythmic

Reference / Resuscitation Council (UK), reproduced with permission.

Adult basic life support

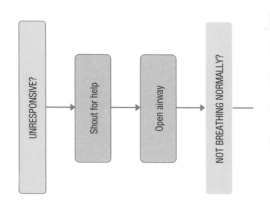

UNRESPONSIVE? → Shout for help → Open airway → NOT BREATHING NORMALLY?

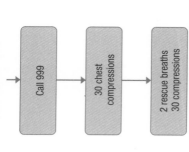

Call 999

30 chest compressions

2 rescue breaths 30 compressions

Reference / Resuscitation Council (UK) (2005) *Resuscitation Guidelines 2005*. London: Resuscitation Council (UK), p. 10. Reproduced with permission.

Paediatric advanced life support

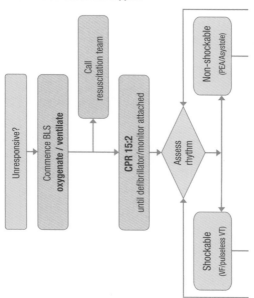

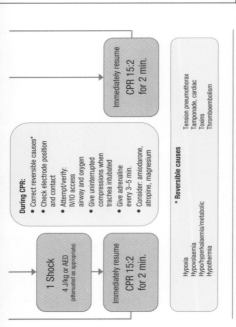

During CPR:
- Correct reversible causes*
- Check electrode position and contact
- Attempt/verify:
  IV/IO access
  airway and oxygen
- Give uninterrupted compressions when trachea intubated
- Give adrenaline every 3–5 min.
- Consider: amiodarone, atropine, magnesium

1 Shock
4 J/kg or AED
(attenuated as appropriate)

Immediately resume CPR 15:2 for 2 min.

Immediately resume CPR 15:2 for 2 min.

* Reversible causes

Hypoxia
Hypovolaemia
Hypo/hyperkalaemia/metabolic
Hypothermia

Tension pneumothorax
Tamponade, cardiac
Toxins
Thromboembolism

Reference / Resuscitation Council (UK) (2005) *Resuscitation Guidelines 2005*. London: Resuscitation Council (UK), p. 86. Reproduced with permission.

Adult advanced life support algorithm

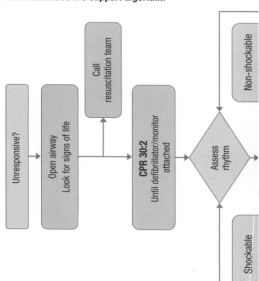

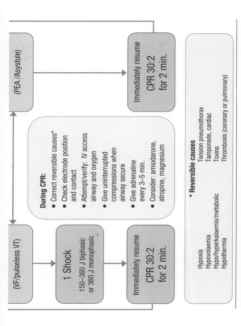

During CPR:
- Correct reversible causes*
- Check electrode position and contact
- Attempt/verify: IV access airway and oxygen
- Give uninterrupted compressions when airway secure
- Give adrenaline every 3–5 min.
- Consider: amiodarone, atropine, magnesium

(VF/pulseless VT)

1 Shock
150–360 J biphasic
or 360 J monophasic

Immediately resume
CPR 30:2
for 2 min.

(PEA /Asystole)

Immediately resume
CPR 30:2
for 2 min.

* **Reversible causes**

Hypoxia	Tension pneumothorax
Hypovolaemia	Tamponade, cardiac
Hypo/hyperkalaemia/metabolic	Toxins
Hypothermia	Thrombosis (coronary or pulmonary)

Reference / Resuscitation Council (UK) (2005) *Resuscitation Guidelines 2005*. London: Resuscitation Council (UK), p. 42. Reproduced with permission.

Wound care

Factors that inhibit healing

GENERAL FACTORS	LOCAL FACTORS
• Age	• Wound management practices
• Underlying disease	• Hydration of wound
• Vascularity	• Temperature of wound
• Nutritional status	• Pressure, friction, shearing forces
• Obesity	• Foreign bodies
• Disorders of sensation/ movement	• Infection
• Drug therapy	
• Psychological state	
• Radiation therapy	

Reference / Carville, K. (2005) *Wound Care Manual*, 5th edn. Perth, Australia: Silver Chain Foundation, p. 39. Reproduced with permission.

Wound colour—Chronic wounds

COLOUR	POTENTIAL MEANING	ACTION
Pink	Epithelialising	Protect
Red	Granulating	Protect
Yellow	Sloughy	Clean
Green	Infected	Clean
Black	Necrotic	Debride

Wound assessment

Following a holistic assessment of the patient, the wound is assessed for:

- Type of healing
- Tissue loss
- Clinical appearance
- Location
- Measurement dimensions
- Exudation
- Surrounding skin
- Pain
- Wound infection
- Psychological implications

Reference / Carville, K. (2005) *Wound Care Manual*, 5th edn. Perth, Australia: Silver Chain Foundation, p. 49. Reproduced with permission.

Calculation of ankle/brachial pressure index (ABPI)

The ankle/brachial pressure index is a Doppler measurement which helps to determine the degree of arterial or venous disease in the leg.

To calculate the ABPI, divide the ankle systolic pressure by the brachial systolic pressure:

$$\frac{\text{Ankle systolic pressure}}{\text{Brachial systolic pressure}} = \text{ABPI}$$

Normal	0.8 to 1.2
Claudiant	0.5 to 0.8
Ischaemic	<0.5
Calcified	>1.2

Ankle/brachial pressure index

<0.5	0.5–0.7	0.7–0.8
Arterial ulcer	Mixed arterial-venous ulcer	
>0.9	>1.2	
Venous ulcer	Possible calcified vessels	

Reference / Carville, K. (2005) *Wound Care Manual*, 5th edn. Perth, Australia: Silver Chain Foundation, p. 96. Reproduced with permission.

Some wound-care products

PRODUCT	ACTION	TYPE OF WOUND
FOAM	• Absorbs, insulates • Promotes autolysis of devitalised tissue	• Needing absorption • Needing protection
HYDROGELS	• Retains moisture, rehydrates • Promotes autolysis of devitalised tissue • Cools surface of wound • Are oxygen permeable	• Needing hydration • Needing autolysis *Note: Not highly exudating*
ALGINATES	• Forms hydrophilic gel when in contact with wound exudate • Facilitates debridement and rehydration of dead tissue	• Cavities • Sinuses • Infected • Needing debridement *Note: Not dry wounds*
TRANSPARENT FILMS	• Promotes epithelialisation • Creates moist environment • Protects from friction	• Needing protection • Needing hydration *Note: Not exudating; caution fragile skin*

PRODUCT	ACTION	TYPE OF WOUND
HYDROCOLLOIDS	• Polymers interact with wound exudate and become gelatinous mass • Protect wounds • Maintain moisture • Waterproof barrier • Promote autolysis of devitalised tissue	• Needing protection • Needing hydration • Needing autolysis *Note Not infected; not involving bone*
SILVERS	• Converts into an ionic form to produce antimicrobial effect • Antimicrobial efficacy of dressing determined by the concentration of silver—needs moisture for silver to be released	• Moderate to heavily exudating • Colonised

In all wound-care products used, it is the responsibility of the nurse to ensure that manufacturers' instructions are followed.

Reference / Adapted from Queensland Government Queensland Health (2004) *Pressure Ulcer Prevention and Management Resource Guideline*. Brisbane: Queensland Health, pp. 46–51. Reproduced with permission.

Documentation

■ GENERAL POINTS

Things to consider

- Check you have the correct patient charts.
- Ensure that what you write is accurate.
- Focus your documentation on the patient.
- Document relevant information only.
- Be objective.
- Document contemporaneously.
- Avoid documenting in advance.
- Don't document on behalf of somebody else.
- Write legibly.
- Use pen (black ink).
- Don't transcribe.
- Use only accepted abbreviations.
- Include a time and a date.
- Identify yourself with a signature and designation.

If an error occurs in documentation

- Rule neatly through the error.
- Don't use correction fluid (white-out) or scribble out the error.
- Write the correction beside or above the mistake.
- The correction should be signed and dated by the person making it.

Writing with SOAPIE

S =	Subjective	What the patient/significant other verbalises
O =	Objective	Data that is measured and observed
A =	Assessment	What is diagnosed from the data gathered
P =	Planning	What care has been planned
I =	Implementation	What care has been implemented
E =	Evaluation	What the outcomes are

Writing with PIE

P = Problem
I = Implementation
E = Evaluation

■ TIPS WITH VERBAL HANDOVERS

Have your essential information prepared before you begin, and include:

Any changes in the patient's/family's situation that is relevant

Normal parameters that have deviated

Doctor rounds—changes in patient's management, any new plans of treatment

Objective (such as vital signs) and subjective data that are relevant

Vicious statements, gossip and personal opinions to be avoided

Education that you have given to the patient/family

Relevant and priority care for the next shift

■ NURSING PROCESS

The nursing process provides a framework for organising nursing care.

The steps are:
- Assessment: Details of the patient assessment and problem identification.
- Planning: A plan of action is developed which includes key activities:
  — setting priorities
  — establishing goals
  — determining nursing interventions
  — documenting nursing care plan
- Implementation: The 'doing' of the plan.
- Evaluation: Making an assessment of the effectiveness of the plan and whether or not changes need to be made.

This process should be ongoing throughout a nurse's day and all steps of the plan need to be documented.

Reference / Adapted from Richards, A. and Edwards, S. (2008) *A Nurse's Survival Guide to the Ward*, 2nd edn. Oxford, England: Churchill Livingstone, pp. 24–5. Reproduced with permission from Elsevier.

General abbreviations

Note *Any abbreviations used should be accepted within your health care organisation prior to use.*

ABG	arterial blood gas
ADL	activities of daily living
AMI	acute myocardial infarction
ARDS	acute respiratory distress syndrome
bid	12 hourly/twice a day
BO	bowels open
Bx	biopsy
Ca	cancer
CAD	coronary artery disease
CCF	congestive cardiac failure
CHD	congenital heart disease
CHF	congestive heart failure
COAD	chronic obstructive airways disease
COPD	chronic obstructive pulmonary disease
CPR	cardio pulmonary resuscitation
CVA	cerebral vascular accident
CVP	central venous pressure
CWMS	colour, warmth, movement, sensation
CXR	chest X-ray
d	day
D	dose
DOB	date of birth
DVT	deep venous thrombosis
ECG	electrocardiogram
FBC	full blood count
FUO	fever of unknown origin
HACC	home and community care

HNPU	has not passed urine
HR	heart rate
Hx	history
ICC	intercostal catheter
IDC	indwelling catheter
IHD	ischaemic heart disease
IVC	intravenous catheter/cannula
IVT	intravenous therapy
JVP	jugular venous pressure
LFT	liver function test
MCS	microscopic culture sensitivity
MI	myocardial infarction
MRSA	multiple/methicillin resistant *Staphylococcus aureus*
MSA	mental state assessment
MSE	Mental state examination
MSU	mid stream urine
MVA	motor vehicle accident
NAD	nil abnormalities detected
NBM	nil by mouth
NGT	naso gastric tube
NIDDM	non-insulin dependent diabetes mellitus (better to use Type 2 DM)
NKA	no known allergies
NOF	neck of femur
O_2	oxygen
Obs	observation
OE	on examination
OR	operating room
ORIF	open reduction and internal fixation
OT	occupational therapy/operating theatre
PAC	pressure area care

PCA	patient controlled analgesia
PD	patient diagnosis/peritoneal dialysis/provisional diagnosis
PE	physical examination/pulmonary embolus
PEG	percutaneous endoscopic gastronomy tube
PICC	peripherally inserted central catheter
PND	paroxysmal nocturnal dyspnoea/postnatal depression
POP	plaster of Paris
PUO	pyrexia unknown origin
PU	passed urine
PVD	peripheral vascular disease
RO	removal of
RLL	right lower lobe
ROM	range of motion
RR	respiratory rate
SI	international system of units
SOB	shortness of breath
SSRI	selective serotonin reuptake inhibitor
Staph	staphylococcus
TAH	total abdominal hysterectomy
TIA	transient ischaemic attack
TPN	total parental nutrition
TPR	temperature, pulse, respiration
Tx	treatment
UA	urinalysis
URTI	upper respiratory tract infection
UTI	urinary tract infection
UWSD	under water sealed drainage
WBC	white blood cell
Wt	weight
yo	years old

Useful www sites

www.jr2.ox.ac.uk/Bandolier
Bandolier: an evidence based website

www.baccn.org.uk
British Association of Critical Care Nurses

www.bnf.org
British National Formulary (BNF)

www.cochrane.org
Cochrane Library

www.cdna-online.org.uk
Community and District Nursing Association (UK)

www.emedicine.com
e-medicine: emergency medicine articles

www.joannabriggs.edu.au
The Joanna Briggs Institute for Evidence Based Nursing and Midwifery

www.amicus-mhna.org
Mental Health Nurses Association

www.nice.org.uk
The National Institute of Health and Clinical Excellence

www.nmc-uk.org
Nursing and Midwifery Council (UK)

www.nursing-portal.com
Nursing Portal: Links provided to quality nursing websites.

www.practicenursing.co.uk
Practice Nursing

www.resus.org.uk
Resuscitation Council (UK)

www.rcn.org.uk
Royal College of Nursing

www.dh.gov.uk
UK Department of Health

www.mhra.gov.uk
UK Medicines and Healthcare Products Regulation Agency

Time management grid

To organise your day, fill out the grid at the beginning of the shift, recording what is due for each client for each hour that you are at work.

Patient name & bed number	What is due Time in hours			

What is due Time in hours					

Other things to remember

Important phone numbers and email addresses

NAME	PHONE NO.	EMAIL